Wasim Pathan

Zygomatic and Pterygoid Implants

Wasim Pathan

Zygomatic and Pterygoid Implants

A Boon to Atrophic Maxilla

LAP LAMBERT Academic Publishing

Publisher:
LAP LAMBERT Academic Publishing
is a trademark of
International Book Market Service Ltd., member of OmniScriptum Publishing Group
17 Meldrum Street, Beau Bassin 71504, Mauritius

ISBN: 978-3-659-69529-2

TOC

INTRODUCTION..01

DEFINITIONS…………........…………07

HISTORY OF IMPLANTS …........……..11

CLASSIFICATION OF IMPLANTS…………………........……14

DENTAL IMPLANT COMPONENTS…………........……..19

ZYGOMATIC IMPLANTS ……........……28

PTERYGOID IMPLANT ……..............…44

SURGICAL PROCEDURE …..........…..62

SUMMARY AND CONCLUSION ……………........…..72

BIBLIOGRAPHY……………........………75

INTRODUCTION

The use of dental implants has evolved significantly in the past decade. Once a rarely used procedures today is a mainstream clinical activity. The development and understanding of endosseous implants have led to high success rates and better acceptance of these implants.

An endosseous implant is currently the closest material or things available to natural tooth. Clinicians have been trying from time immemorial to provide their patients with results that are both aesthetically, as well as functionally, if not natural, then closest to it.

Implant therapy offers many advantages over conventional fixed or removable treatment options and in many cases is the treatment of choice.

However, its potential benefits and high success rateshave led to the procedure sometimes being incorrectly used, with unfortunate outcomes. A wide range of components is low available from many different manufacturers, and the technique is developing its own jargon.

Implants have long fascinated clinicians with the immense possibilities they bring with them in terms of results. Thus, a huge number of materials, types, techniques, etc have been developed with implants.

Severely resorbed edentulous maxillae present very complex problems for the surgeon and the clinician.

Lack of internal osseous stimulation and non-physiologic crestal bone loading results in continued resorption of an already atrophic edentulous maxilla. The end result is an inability to use a conventional full denture prosthesis. In 1999 **Dr. Per-Ingvar Branemark** and colleagues introduced the zygoma implant (P-I Branemark, personal communication, 1999).

The availability of the zygoma implant has provided a viable alternative for treatment of patients with extreme resorption of the edentulous maxilla or large pneumatized maxillary sinuses.[1,2] Before the introduction of this fixture, implant supported or retained fixed or removable prostheses in the atrophic maxilla could only be considered after extensive ridge preparation.

Before the introduction of this fixture, implant supported or retained fixed or removable prosthesis in the atrophic maxilla could only be considered after extensive ridge preparation.

This preparation usually included major autologous bone grafting, prolonged treatment times, long-term inability to wear any prosthesis, and a higher failure rate for conventional implants placed in large bone grafts.

In 1999 **Dr. Per-Ingvar Branemark** and colleagues introduced the zygoma implant (P-I Brånemark, personal communication, 1999). In their initial study over a 10-year period, 110 implants were placed. Each patient had an additional two to four conventional implants placed in the anterior maxilla, which was restored with cross arch stabilization. Of the zygoma fixtures placed and restored in the initial study, only two were lost in the first year of occlusal loading, and three failed in the subsequent 8 years for a long term success rate of >95%.

The zygoma implant is an extended-length (30–52.5 mm) machined titanium fixture that is placed through the crestal (slightly palatal) aspect of the resorbed posterior maxilla trans-antrally into the compact bone of the zygoma. In addition to two to four conventional fixtures in the anterior maxilla, initial stability of this elongated fixture is assured by its contact with four osseous cortices[3 4 5.]

1. At the ridge crest

2. The sinus floor

3. The roof of the maxillary sinus

4. The superior border of the zygoma

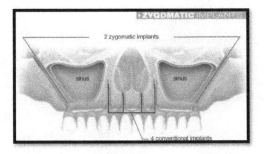 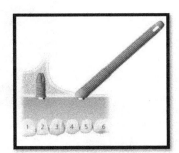

The zygoma implant provides posterior maxillary anchorage when the existing osseous structures do not allow standard implant placement. The alternative in this situation includes bone graft augmentation (sinus lifts and onlay grafts) with their attendant costs, discomfort, prolonged treatment times, and higher complication rates. The zygoma fixture is suggested in the following circumstances:

- When full maxillary edentulism is accompanied by advanced posterior resorption that would otherwise require grafting. At least two and preferably four anterior standard implants are needed in combination with bilateral zygoma implants.

- In partial or incomplete maxillectomy patients when additional implants can be placed in other sites such as the piriform sinus, orbital rims, palatal shelves, or pterygoid plates to support cross-arch stabilization.

The maxillary tuberosity is often well developed but is made of bone that is too spongy to provide predictable osseointegration.

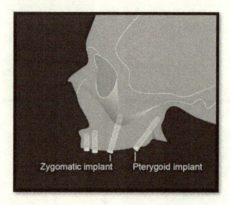

The tuberosity rests against an extremely dense mass of bone formed by the pterygoid process and the vertical point of the palatine bone.

Branemark used the Tuberosity as early as 1975, **Jean-Francois Tulasne** placed the first implant at the suggestion of **Paul Tessier** (1985)

The Branemark System has demonstrated high success rates for implants placed in completely edentulous jaws since its introduction to clinical dentistry in 1965. **Adell** and coworkers demonstrated 15 years of functional and successful results in the treatment of edentulous jaws; however, the majority of implants in the maxilla were placed anterior to the maxillary antrum. Other researchers have also documented the success of the Brånemark implant system. According to **Zarb et al**, the posterior maxilla is the most difficult and problematic intraoral area for treatment with osseointegrated implants.

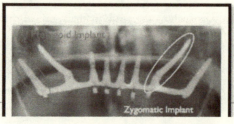

Bone in pterygoid area is cortical in nature, and hence it is very strong and rigid that an implant in that region can be loaded easily. Pterygoid implant are the implants located in 2nd molar area of the upper jaw. Major advantage of this implant is flapless technique which lowers down the chances of swelling or bleeding post operatively. No sinus lift and no bone grafts has to be done while using this implant.

Throughout literature, several terms are being used to describe pterygoid implant. The terms "pterygoid implant", "pterygomaxillary implants" and "tuberosity implants" are used interchangeably.

Pterygoid implants have been defined by the Glossary of Oral and Maxillofacial Implants (GOMI) as "implant placement through the maxillary tuberosity and into the pterygoid plate".

Pterygoid implants originate in the tuberosity and engage in the dense bone of the pterygoid plates and palatine bone.

Reiser performed a cadaver study analysing through which bony structures, implants placed in the pterygomaxillary region are being supported. In cases with sufficient bone quality and quantity of the tuberosity, the implant can be placed entirely within the tuberosity.

It was previously thought that the pterygomaxillary area was inoperable and not suited for implants because of large fatty marrow spaces, limited trabecular bone, and the rare presence of cortical bone covering the alveolus. Because of these anatomic factors and some biomechanical factors, one would expect the success rate for implants placed into the posterior maxilla to be lower than that for other locations. In 1991, **Reiger** recommended using a larger number of implants in the posterior maxilla to compensate for the decreased predictability for osseointegration in that area. **Langer et al** recommended the use of wider diameter implants to obtain a greater surface area for bone contact. Bone-graft procedures, such as sinus lifts and onlay grafts, were also introduced to address some of these anatomic conditions, but these procedures require a longer healing period and may present other complications.

In addition, there is a risk of morbidity at the donor site with autogenous bone grafting procedures. **Jaffin** and **Berman** reported on implants used specifically in the maxillary posterior and noted a higher failure rate related to Type IV bone. **Schnitman** 20 demonstrated that the posterior maxilla was the least successful area for osseointegration to occur. In his report, only 72% of implants placed in the posterior maxilla achieved osseointegration. Force factors are another variable affecting the long-term stability of implants, particularly in the posterior region. The magnitude of occlusal load is larger in the molar region than in the anterior region. Masticatory forces of 155 N have been reported in the incisor region, with comparative forces of 288 N and 565 N in the premolar and molar regions, respectively. In parafunction, these forces can be as much as 3 times the normal masticatory forces, which would apply significant stress to the bone-implant interface and the component hardware. Posterior cantilevers on implant prostheses produce complications, including screw fracture, prosthesis fracture, bone loss, and loss of osseointegration.

Improving biomechanical stability and load distribution by means of non -cantilevered, bone-anchored restorations should enhance the long-term prognosis of implant restorations in the posterior maxilla.

DEFINITIONS

DENTAL IMPLANT

- A prosthetic device made of alloplastic material(s) implanted into the oral tissues beneath the mucosal or/and periosteal layer, and on/or within the bone to provide retention and support for a fixed or removable dental prosthesis; a substance that is placed into or/and upon the jaw bone to support a fixed or removable dental prosthesis - GPT

- The portion of an implant that provides support for the dental implant abutment(s) through adaptation upon with in or through the bone usage.

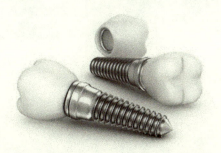

ZYGOMZTIC IMPLANT

- Zygomatic implants are long screw-shaped implants which are developed as an alternative to bone grafting and sinus augmentation for resorbed, atrophic or fractured maxillae. These were first described by **Branemark** in 1998.

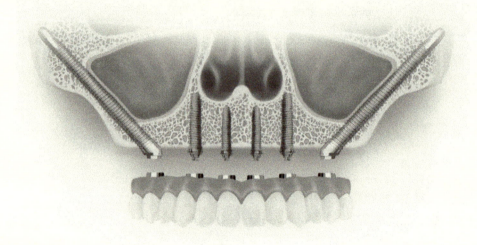

PTERYGOID IMPLANT

Throughout literature, several terms are being used to describe **Pterygoid implants**. The terms "pterygoid implants", "pterygomaxillary implants" and "tuberosity implants" are used interchangeably.

"Pterygoid implants" have been defined by the Glossary of Oral and Maxillofacial Implants (GOMI) as "implant placement through the maxillary tuberosity and into the pterygoid plate".

There are significant differences between pterygoid and tuberosity implants including the following:

- Pterygoid implants originate in the tuberosity and engage in the dense bone of the pterygoid plates and palatine bone
- Tuberosity implants originate in the maxillary alveolar process and can occasionally anchor in the pyramidal process. The bone quality in this region is mainly composed of type III or IV cancellous bone.

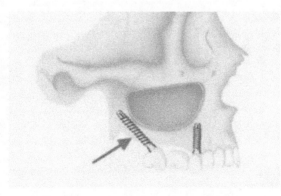

Reiser performed a cadaver study analyzing through which bony structures implants placed in the pterygomaxillary region are being supported. In cases with sufficient bone quality and quantity of the tuberosity, the implant can be placed entirely within the tuberosity.

HISTORY OF IMPLANTS

Replacement of lost dentition has been traced to ancient Egyptian and South American civilizations. In ancient Egyptian writings implanted animal and carved ivory teeth were the oldest examples of primitive implantology. In eighteenth and nineteenth century England and colonial America, poor individuals sold their teeth for extraction and transplantation to wealthy recipients who used these teeth to replace their missing teeth. The clinical outcomes of these transplanted dentitions were either ankylosis or root resorption.

Continued research prolonged allotransplant survival but did not appreciably improve predictability. In 1809 Maggiolo placed an immediate single-stage gold implant in a fresh extraction site with the coronal aspect of the fixture protruding just above the gingiva. The postoperative complications included severe pain and gingival inflammation. Since then various implant materials were used ranging from roughened lead roots holding a platinum post to tubes of gold and iridium.

Adams in 1937 patented a submergible threaded cylindrical implant with a ball head screwed to the root for retention for an overdenture in a fashion similar to that done today. Up to this point implant success was marginal with a maximum longevity of only a few years.

Strock placed the first long-term endosseous implant at Harvard in 1938. This implant was a threaded cobalt-chrome-molybdenum screw with a cone shaped head for the cementation of a jacket crown. The implant remained stable and asymptomatic until 1955, at which time the patient died in a car accident. Strock wrote, "The histological sections of implants in the dog study showed remarkable complete tolerance of the dental implant and the pathologist report so indicated to our gratification." Strock demonstrated for the first time that metallic endosteal dental implants were tolerated in humans, with a survival rate of upto 17 years.

Due to inadequate alveolar bone height in certain sites of the jaws, subperiosteal implants were developed. In 1943 Dahl placed a metal structure on the maxillary alveolar crest with four projecting posts. Multiple variations to this initial design were fabricated but these devices often resulted in wound dehiscence.

Blade implants were introduced by Linkow and by Roberts and Roberts. There were numerous configurations with broad applications, and the implants became the most widely used device in implantology in the United States and abroad.

A two-staged threaded titanium root form implant was first presented in North America by Branemark in 1978. He showed that titanium oculars, placed in the femurs of rabbits, osseointegrated in the femurs of rabbits after a period of healing. Two-staged titanium implants were first placed in patients in 1965 and studies showed prolonged survival, freestanding function, bone maintenance, and significant improvement in benefit-to-risk ratio over all previous implants.

This breakthrough has revolutionized maxillofacial reconstruction. Subsequently, various implant designs have been manufactured and research in implantology has grown exponentially. The frontiers of implantology are rapidly being advanced and aesthetics continue to be an integral part of this progress.

Extensive work by the Swedish orthopaedic surgeon Per Ingvar Branemark led to the discovery that commercially pure titanium, when placed in a suitably prepared site in the bone, could become fixed in place due to a close bond that developed between the two, a phenomenon that he later described as osseointegration .

This state has anatomical and functional dimensions, as it requires both a close contact between the implant and surrounding healthy bone and the ability to transmit functional loads over an extended period without deleterious effects either systemically or in the adjacent tissues.

OI is not defined in terms of the extent of the bone-implant contact, provided that functional requirements are met and the tissues are healthy. Many of the factors that predispose to the development of OI are now known, and where these exist a successful outcome will probably follow the placing of a suitable implant.

Similarly, failure is more likely where factors known to predispose to an unsuccessful outcome exist. Occasionally, implants fail for no apparent reason, sometimes in groups in one patient - the so-called 'cluster phenomenon'. It is therefore important to advise patients that a satisfactory outcome cannot be guaranteed.

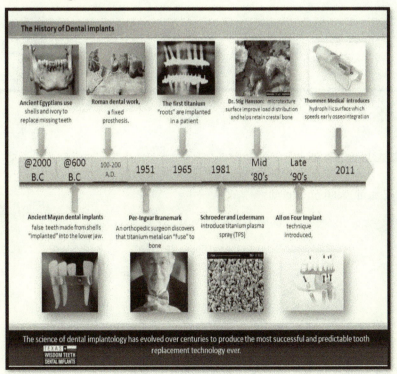

The History of Dental Implants

Ancient Egyptians use shells and ivory to replace missing teeth	Roman dental work, a fixed prosthesis.	The first titanium "roots" are implanted in a patient	Dr. Stig Hansson: microtexture surface improve load distribution and helps retain crestal bone	Thommen Medical introduces hydrophilic surface which speeds early osseointegration

| @2000 B.C | @600 B.C | 100-200 A.D. | 1951 | 1965 | 1981 | Mid '80's | Late '90's | 2011 |

| Ancient Mayan dental implants false teeth made from shells "implanted" into the lower jaw. | Per-Ingvar Branemark An orthopedic surgeon discovers that titanium metal can "fuse" to bone | Schroeder and Ledermann introduce titanium plasma spray (TPS) | All on Four Implant technique introduced, |

The science of dental implantology has evolved over centuries to produce the most successful and predictable tooth replacement technology ever.

TEXAS WISDOM TEETH DENTAL IMPLANTS

CLASSIFICATION OF IMPLANTS

Based on position of implants:-

- Sub-periosteal implant
- Endosteal or Endosseous implant
  - ➢ Plate-form implant
  - ➢ Root-form implant
- Transosseous implant
- Intramucosal implant

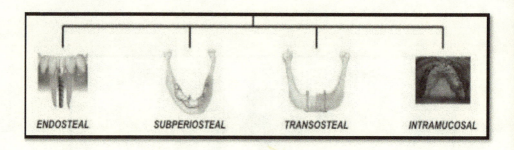

ENDOSTEAL   SUBPERIOSTEAL   TRANSOSTEAL   INTRAMUCOSAL

Based on shape and form:-

A. Post or root form implants

- Solid Tapering Types
- Solid Cylinder Types
- Pin Types
- Screw Shaped
- Basket Design
- Hollow Cylinder Design

B. Blade implants

- Conventional Blade Design
- Vented Blade Design

Based on surface characteristics:-

- Titanium plasma-sprayed coating
- Sand blasting-surface etching
- Laser induced surface roughening
- Hydroxyapatite coating

Based on surface of implant body:-

- Smooth
- Machined
- Textured
- Coated

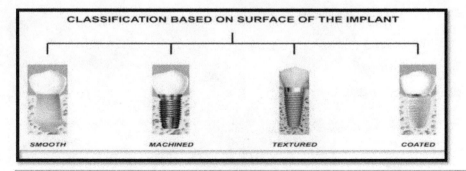

Based on implant tissue interface:-

- Osseointegration
- Fibrointegration

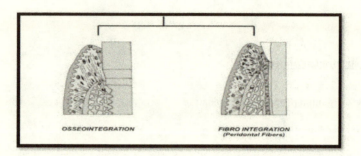

Based on foundation:-

- Implant supported
- Implant assisted

Based on mode of retention of prosthesis:-

- Fixed
- Removable

Based on various systems:-

- Branemark implant system

- International team for oral implant

- Implant innovations system

- Astra dental implant system

- Endosteal hollow basket system

Depending on the materials used

1. METALLIC IMPLANTS

- Titanium

- Cobalt chromium molybdenum alloy- Titanium aluminum vanadium

- Cobalt chromium molybdenum

- Stainless steel

- Zirconium

- Tantalum

- Gold

- Platinum

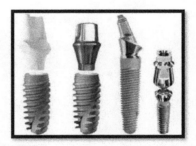

Fig. Metallic Implants

2. NON – METALLIC IMPLANTS

- Ceramics

- Carbon

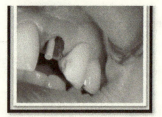 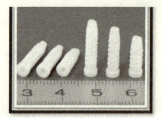

Fig. Non Metallic Implants

Depending On Their Reaction With Bone

Based on the ability of implant to stimulate bone formation

3. Bio active

  - Hydroxyapatite

  - Tri Calcium Phosphate

  - Calcium Phosphate

4. Bio inert

  • Metals

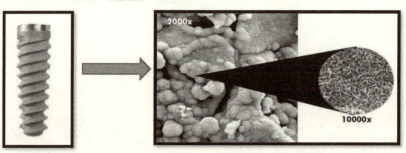

DENTAL IMPLANT COMPONENTS

- **IMPLANT BODY**

  - ➤ Often referred to as an implant

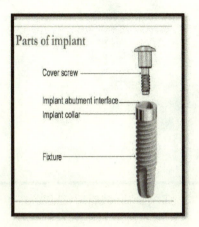

- **COVER SCREW**

  - ➤ Prevents bone ingress in the implant head

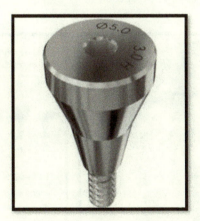

- **TRANSMUCOSAL ABUTMENT (TMA)**

    - Links the implant body to the mouth. May be pre-manufactured or custom formed

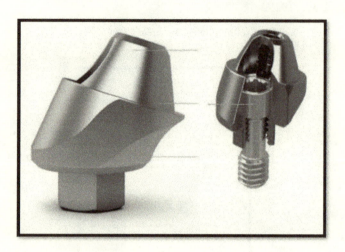

- **HEALING ABUTMENT**

    - Placed temporarily on the implant body to maintain patency of the mucosal penetration

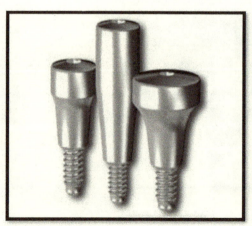
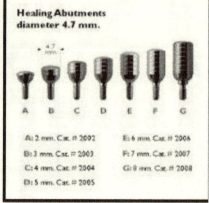

- **IMPRESSION COPING**

  ➤ Used to transfer the location of the implant body or abutment to a

  dental cast

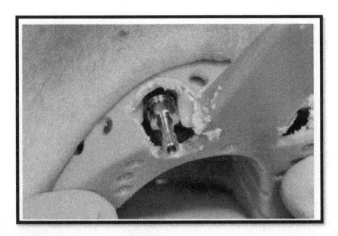

- **LABORATORY ANALOGUE**

  ➤ A base metal replica of the implant body, or a pre-manufactured

  abutment

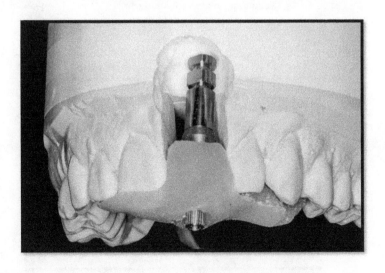

- **GOLD CYLINDER**

  ➢ Pre-manufactured to fit an abutment and form part of a prosthesis

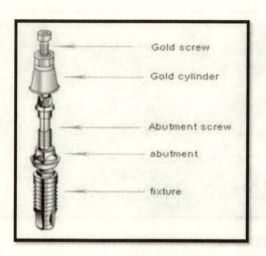

- **HEALING CAPS**

  ➢ Temporary covers for abutmets

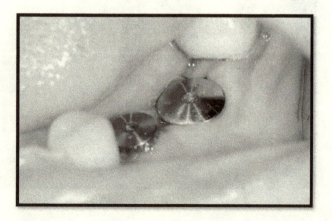

INDICATIONS

1. Edentulous patient

2. Partially edentulous patient with history of difficulty in wearing R.P.D.

3. Patient requiring long span F.P.D. treatment

4. Patient who refuses wearing a removable prosthesis

5. Patient with severe changes in C.D. bearing tissues

6. Poor oral muscular coordination

7. Parafunctional habits that compromise prosthesis stability

8. Unrealistic patient expectation for complete denture

9. Hyperactive gag reflex

10. Patient psychologically against removable prosthesis

11. Unfavourable number and location of abutments

12. Single tooth loss, avoid preparation of sound teeth

CONTRAINDICATIONS

ABSOLUTE

1.   High dose irradiated patient

2.   Patient with psychiatric problems

3.   Systemic hematologic disorders

RELATIVE

1.   Pathology of hard or soft tissue

2.   Recent extraction site

3.   Patient with drug, alcohol, or chewing tobacco

4.   Low dose irradiated patient

TREATMENT PLANNING

Treatment with dental implants has evolved from earlier procedures to a mainstream clinical activity. However, its potential benefits and high success rates have led to the procedure sometimes being incorrectly used, with unfortunate outcomes. A wide range of components is now available from many different manufacturers.

GENERAL TREATMENT DECISIONS

Treatment with dental implants has considerably extended the range of care that we can offer our patients. However, despite its applications in new areas such as maxillofacial prosthodontics, the anchoring of hearing aids and in orthodontic therapy, it is principally used for prosthodontic rehabilitation. If the potential benefits of such uses are to be maximized, then it is essential that implant treatment should be selected on a logical basis.

GATHERING INFORMATION AND TREATMENT PLANNING

Treatment should not be based on hope, be it in the mind of the surgeon or the patient, but rather on accurate information, an understanding of the patient's problems, recognition of suitable treatment alternatives and the agreed selection of the one most appropriate to their needs. This may not necessarily be the most complex procedure or involve the use of dental implants. Their use is most likely to succeed where it has been selected on a sound basis.

IMPLANT SURGERY

The correct insertion of dental implants is essential for their optimal utilization and involves far more than merely the surgical creation of an intra-bony defect and insertion of the implant body. The technique must involve appropriate planning and consultation by the dental team, even where the surgeon and prosthodontist are the same individual. While an integrated dental implant is essential for success, it is of little use if it is inappropriately located.

THE EDENTULOUS CASE

While the number of edentulous individuals is falling in many countries, those that remain are often oral cripples. It was for this reason that treatment of such patients was one of the priorities for the early pioneers of dental implantology. The procedure can bring enormous benefits to such patients but must be set against a background of prosthodontic knowledge; an inadequate prosthesis does not become ideal merely because it is implant stabilized.

THE PARTIALLY EDENTULOUS CASE

The great benefits achievable with implant treatment in the edentulous patient were soon translated into the resolution of specific problems in the partially dentate patient, where they have been shown to be highly effective in appropriate cases. The situation is, however, more complex than in the edentulous case, since there are often several treatment modalities that could be used, while the status of the existing teeth and their supporting structures are additional complications. Dental implants are not an alternative to inadequate oral hygiene or poor treatment planning, and if inserted inappropriately in the partially dentate patient can present a major problem when further teeth are lost.

THE SINGLE-TOOTH SCENARIO

Missing single teeth, especially due to trauma, are not an uncommon problem, which in many cases can be easily solved using traditional restorative techniques. However, there are some situations where this is not technically feasible or produces an inferior result. Recognizing these cases, planning and carrying out appropriate implant-based treatment are discussed in this chapter.

OTHER APPLICATIONS

The ability of osseointegrated interfaces to develop in many locations has led to a wide range of potential applications for dental and skull implants.[32]

PROBLEMS

Treatment with dental implants can be a very complex procedure in terms of planning, execution and management of the complications. Despite the high success rate of the technique, these are not unknown and are best managed by avoidance rather than correction after the event.[32]

ZYGOMATIC IMPLANTS

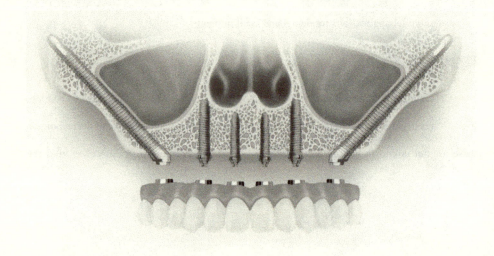

INDICATIONS

While the zygoma implant is most often used in cases of moderate to severe atrophy, it can be considered a valuable procedure for any patient in need of posterior maxillary implant support with or without significant atrophy. The ability to avoid grafting in many patients, along with the continuous use of an interim maxillary prosthesis also makes the zygoma implant approach appealing as a treatment option.

1. Moderate Atrophy

The majority of patients who present with a medium- to long-term history of denture wear will have a moderate degree of atrophy. This category of denture experience constitutes the majority of patients who seek implant therapy to reverse the effects of continuing bone loss and prosthesis instability. Many will be candidates for grafting procedures, such as sinus augmentation or block onlay techniques, as a means of creating additional osseous structure to allow enough support for implants. The ability to avoid such grafting is one of the principal benefits of considering the zygoma implant alternative.

2. Severe Atrophy

Although most of these patients will essentially be graft candidates, there are some who, because of history or physical circumstances, cannot or will not undergo these procedures. A history of consistent graft failure or a systemic compromise that contraindicates grafting are examples of mitigating factors that may require considering an alternative approach such as use of the zygoma implant. Experience to date with these patients is not extensive, but early indications of implant survival are seen as encouraging, even with the most severely compromised maxillae. Prosthesis design for the severely atrophic maxilla with implant support may be influenced by the relative size disparity between the two jaws. Most such atrophy results in an undersized maxilla relative to the corresponding mandible, even in cases where both arches are equally resorbed. Cantilever considerations and implant stress distribution may mandate the use of an overdenture prosthesis rather than a fixed restoration in order to manage occlusal alignment and lateral spacing.

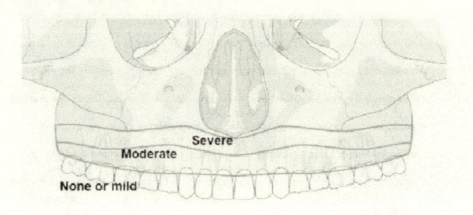

Fig : Image demonstrating mild, moderate and severe atrophy of maxilla

3. Inadequate Posterior Support

Occasionally patients will present with adequate bone for anterior or premaxillary implants but have sinus extensions that eliminate the potential for posterior implants without augmentation. If such grafting is indicated but countermanded by patient request or health considerations, the zygoma approach can be equally effective.

4. Syndromic Patients

Another less frequent indication for the zygoma approach can present in patients with various anodontias from syndromes such as cleidocranial dysostosis or ectodermal dysplasia. Radiographs may show either impacted and unerupted teeth or missing dentition, resulting in growth patterns of the maxilla that are disrupted and minimized. These individuals often present with insufficient bone for adequate numbers of implants and can be difficult to graft because of space or soft tissue limitations. Zygoma implants can be valuable in these instances when combined with conventional fixtures to provide the basis for long-term prosthetic support at a relatively early age.

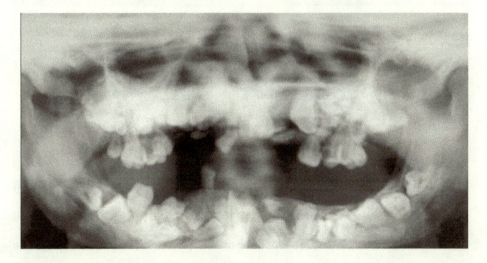

Fig: Image showing O.P.G of the patient suffering from Cleidocranial Dysostosis.

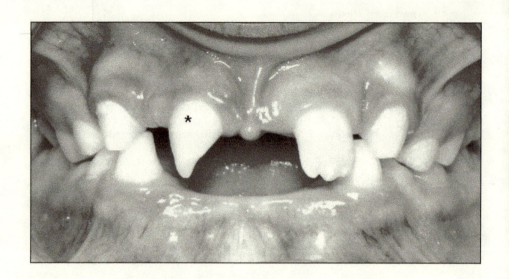

Fig: Image showing dentition affected by Ectodermal Dysplasia.

5. Acquired and Congenital Defects

Maxillary defects created by secondary intervention, such as tumor removal or by trauma, can often be treated with zygoma implant therapy to provide retention for an obturating prosthesis. Similarly, congenital defects such as an unrepaired adult cleft palate (which are increasingly rare owing to early surgical closure) can often be treated with conventional implants in combination with zygoma fixtures to support a removable prosthetic appliance. Situations such as these are rarely the same because of the wide variations in residual soft tissue and bone anatomy, and each case will require careful individual planning to assess the potential for implant placement or zygoma use.

For many, however, the ability to use remote bone anchorage with implants around the defect periphery can create excellent supplemental retentive possibilities for these often large and otherwise poorly supported prosthetic devices.

6. Immediate Loading

Literature citations supporting the possibility of immediate loading of maxillary implants increasingly support this concept[6-9]. The criteria for attempting this approach are generally the same as for immediate loading anywhere in the oral cavity: adequate initial stability, good bone receptor sites, and initial cross-arch splinting with rigid materials. In situations where these criteria can be met, the survival prospects for both conventional and zygoma fixtures appear to be equivalent to the rates attained with the delayed approach. The benefits in patient comfort, convenience, and enhanced function make this a desirable option in appropriately selected cases.

7. Partial Edentulism

The original concept of the zygoma implant, used with anterior implants and cross-arch stabilization, would theoretically not have application for posterior maxillary partial edentulism.

In practice, however, there is potential for using the zygoma implant through the sinus, with additional fixtures on either side, to support a fixed partial denture. This approach has not been thoroughly investigated, and clinical trials do not provide enough longevity to make a definitive statement regarding the efficacy of this technique. Being able to gain strong intermediate support through sinus areas that would otherwise have to be grafted does have enough merit, however, to warrant further investigation.[33]

CONTRAINDICATIONS

1. Other than the most obvious contraindications, such as systemic compromise or sinus disease, there are only two specific situations that would complicate the use of the zygoma implant or make it unnecessary.

2. First, where adequate maxillary bone exists for implant placement in numbers and positions to support a prosthetic appliance, the zygoma implant is not needed.

3. The second situation is where there is not enough premaxillary support for at least two stable implants with good potential longevity. Differential diagnosis, infact, often depends more on the volume and condition of anterior bone than existing posterior anatomy to determine whether some edentulous patients may be candidates for this procedure. In such instances, bone-grafting procedures should be considered preprosthetically, to create an adequate osseous base for effective cross-arch stabilization.[33]

THE SURGICAL PROCEDURE

Surgery for zygoma implant placement is best performed using deep intravenous sedation or a general anesthetic. Local anesthesia with vestibular infiltration, nerve blocks, and percutaneous blocks or infiltration lateral and superior to the zygomatic notch just lateral to the orbital rim should be administered. Bilateral inferior alveolar nerve blocks are also helpful if the procedure is performed with sedation because significant retraction of the tongue, lower lip, and mandible are needed to ensure adequate access for the procedure.

A crestal incision, placed slightly to the palatal aspect of the ridge in the first molar–second bicuspid region is made from the right- to left- tuberosity regions with bilateral releasing incisions at the incision ends. A releasing incision at the maxillary midline is also helpful for flap development and retraction. The lateral maxilla is exposed by elevating full thickness mucoperiosteal flaps sufficient to visualize the zygomatic buttress from ridge crest to the superior surface of the zygoma at the zygomatic notch, just lateral to the orbit. The anterior maxilla is exposed to the piriform rims to avoid tearing the flap during retraction and to allow placement of conventional anterior maxillary implants. The entire lateral surface of the zygomatic buttress is exposed using a palpating finger extraorally at the zygomatic notch to ensure that the dissection is not directed into the orbital floor.

During the dissection, the infraorbital nerve should be identified and protected. A fissure bur, usually a 703 or 702, in a straight surgical handpiece is used to make a "slot" exposure vertically in the lateral wall of the sinus near the height of the zygomatic buttress. The slot should parallel the planned course of the zygoma implant just medial to the lateral sinus wall. The slot should extend from near the sinus floor at the planned site of implant placement superiorly to near the roof of the sinus.

Preparation of the slot in the sinus wall allows the surgeon to visualize directly the passage of all drill preparations and implant insertion through the lateral sinus. When preparing the slot, the schneiderian membrane in the sinus is removed to allow good visualization and to prevent its interference with site preparation and implant insertion.Ifportions of the membranes are "picked up" by the implant and carried into the implant preparation in the body of the zygoma, they could interfere with osseointegration. A series of long drills are used for incremental preparation of the implant site.

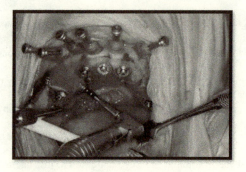

The zygoma implant varies in length from 30 to 52.5 mm.[33] The apical two-thirds of the implant is 4 mm in diameter and the alveolar one-third is 5 mm in diameter. The initial drill is a round bur,which is used to start the implant preparation at the second bicuspid–first molar area as near the crest of the residual alveolar ridge as possible— usually slightly to the palatal aspect. The surgeon must preserve enough bone lateral to the site to fully surround the alveolar portion of the implant. The round bur is directed through the sinus floor and through the lateral sinus superiorly following the axis of the lateral wall slot preparation to the top of the sinus where it indents the site of the preparation in the zygoma body. The slot preparation allows direct visualization of the passage of the drill and the subsequent instrumentation and implant insertion. A custom-designed zygoma retractor with a toe-out tip is kept in position over the zygomatic notch throughout the site preparation to provide good visualization and protect the surrounding anatomy. The retractor also has a midline marker that parallels the site preparation and assists in orientation of the drills in the proper direction. Subsequent drills to complete the preparation are, in sequence, long 2.9 mm diameter twist drills, a 2.9 mm to 3.5 mm pilot drill, and a 3.5 mm twist drill.

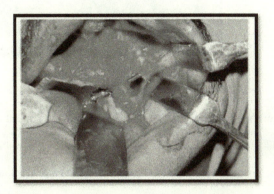

The preparation is carried through the body of the zygoma, through the cortex at the superior border of the zygoma body at the notch. The soft tissues at the superior portion of the preparation are protected by the zygoma retractor. Each fissure bur has incremental markings from 30 to 52.5 mm, which help the surgeon determine the needed implant length. When the preparation is complete, final determination of implant length is made using the zygoma implant depth gauge.[33]

Lastly, if the residual alveolar bone is substantial, a 4 mm twist drill is used to complete the alveolar portion of the preparation. If the residual alveolar bone is spongy, this step is usually eliminated. The zygoma implant has an angulated abutment platform. The 45° angulation allows the platform of the implant to emerge in the same plane as that of the conventional implants that will be placed in the anterior maxilla. Premounted implant carriers are already attached to the zygoma implants for handling of the fixture with the handpiece.

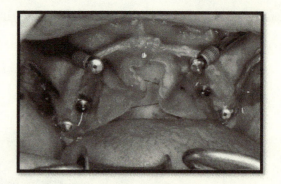

The implant is inserted with copious irrigation, directly visualizing its passage through the lateral sinus through the slot preparation. During insertion, the implant must stay in the same plane as the drills in order to ensure its engagement in the preparation site at the zygoma body. The slot preparation should be extended superiorly far enough to allow visualization of the preparation. When site preparation has been adequately performed, the handpiece will stall when the apical portion of the implant engages 2 to 3 mm of dense zygomatic bone. When this occurs, a manual driver is used to complete implant insertion. Proper angulation of the abutment platform is determined by placing a screwdriver in the implant carrier screw head and seating the implant until the screwdriver is perpendicular to the crest of the edentulous ridge. The implant carrier is removed and a cover screw is placed.

After placement o fthe zygoma implants, two to four regular platform Mark III or Mark IV Nobel Biocare implants are placed in the anterior maxilla. The flaps are repositioned and sutured. The maxillary denture is relieved, hollowed out at the implant emergence sites, and soft-lined with a tissue conditioner. Prior to closure, implant level impressions are made. This allows for fabrication of a rigid bar to be placed at second-stage surgery about 6 months later. The patient's denture prosthesis is relined as often as is necessary over the 6-month osseointegration period.

At second-stage surgery, the cast rigid bar is attached to the implant fixtures, providing immediate cross-arch stabilization. The denture is further hollowed out and relined or a transitional fixed prosthesis is constructed and attached. Four to 6 weeks later, after the soft tissues are healed, impressions are made and the definitive prosthesis is constructed.[33]

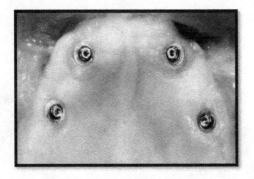

THE PROSTHETIC PROCEDURE

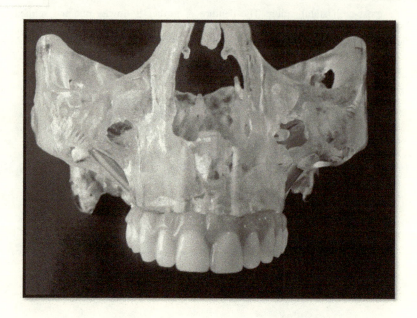

<u>Healing Phase:</u>

Maintenance of the implant is one of the key factor in the completion of the procedure right from stage 1. The existing upper denture can be modified for immediate use thus maintaining the esthetics of the patient. The patient can face difficulty in functions such as chewing along with lesser retention of the denture but the presence of teeth throughout the procedure is far more better in esthetics as compared to no teeth at all.

Protective Splinting:

zygomatic implant when used along with splinting and cross arch stabilization provides excellent strength. It may cause difficulty in maintainance of osseointegration when loaded independently. Following stage II surgery it is important to prevent independent stress transfer from denture base to the individual implant[10.]

To achieve this the following procedure is carried out:

All newly exposed implants with abutments are splinted with a soldered bar within 24 hours. An impression is made immediately after the abutment is delivered. A gold bar of approximately 2 mm in diameter is bent to contour so that it touches a set of gold cylinders attached to the abutment analogs on the cast. With a micro welding device the bar and cylinders can be soldered together and within a short time period a passive protective splint can be fabricated. The bar splint is delivered the next day and the denture is bevelled to allow proper fixation without bar interference. A complete soft liner can be applied to the upper denture to increase comfort and retention. Bar splint is not mandatory if the patient is not wearing an upper denture but in cases were the patient has to wear continuous denture the bar splint should be given[33.]

Final Prosthesis Construction

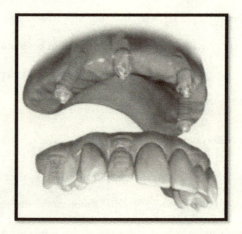

After an adequate healing period of 3-4 weeks, final impressions can be made. Implant-stabilized record bases and wax rims are used to record jaw relations. Try-in is done, and esthetics of the patient is confirmed. For creation of a metal bar structure the putty indexes are made and are hence used to provide a matrix for the same. A second try-in is done for evaluation of passive fit and esthetics followed by denture processing. Screw and screw torques are used to provide complete seating. The bar structures are generally waxed and cast in solid blocks of titanium for excellent passive fit properties. the advantage of milled titanium is that it prevent distortion through the thermocycling phases of veneering. In some situations like high load forces a porcelain fused to metal restoration can be used. This will provide support for the veneering material[33.]

COMPLICATIONS

1. The loss of zygoma implant compromises the posterior anchorage and the cantilever extention may overstress the other components in the first molar region.

2. Correction of this imbalance requires a period of healing at original site followed by replacement of a second implant[33.]

PTERYGOID IMPLANT

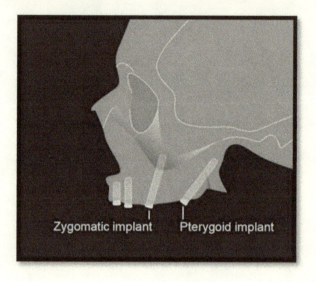

Zygomatic implant   Pterygoid implant

INDICATIONS

1. Maxillary sinus and limited bone quality can be challenging task for the placement for implant in the upper jaw which is edentulous.

2. Patients with similar bone loss levels to those of conventional implants and where patients need less augmentation of bone.

3. It can be done to avoid sinus lift procedure.

However, at present, pterygoid implants have mainly been studied in partial edentulism as a very attractive treatment alternative to sinus lift procedures.

CONTRAINDICATIONS

1. Inadequate amount of bone.

2. Severe bone resorption due to bony disease like osteoporosis

3. Patient on chaemotherapy

4. High dose irradiated patient

5. Patient with psychiatric problems

6. Systemic hematologic disorders

7. Pathology of hard or soft tissues

PTERYGOID IMPLANTS TO SUPPORT A MAXILLARY PROSTHESIS AFTER MAXILLECTOMY

One of the most serious complication after bilateral maxillectomy is esthetic and functional compromise. Surgical implant placement, retention and support of maxillary obturator prosthesis is also challenging in these patients. So as to overcome these problems zygoma implants, pterygoid/ pterygomaxillary implants are the treatment of choice.

MAXILLECTOMY

Maxillectomy or maxillary resection is defined as surgical removal of a part or all of the maxilla[34.] This definition is broad and does not describe the resection in lateral, superior, or posterior extensions. A classification system described by Spiro et al is simple and is popular among surgeons and maxillofacial prosthodontists[35-42]. In this system, adjectives are used to describe the extent of maxillary resection as limited, subtotal, or total. Limited maxillectomy is defined as any maxillary resection that primarily removes one wall of the antrum, usually the floor or the medial wall.

Subtotal maxillectomy is defined as any maxillectomy that removes at least 2 walls, including the floor of the antrum (hard palate) but not the posterior wall.

Total maxillectomy is defined as complete removal of the maxilla, usually involving orbital exenteration. Additional details, such as unilateral or bilateral and the contiguous structures involved, are usually specified along with the classified resection. Obturation of bilateral subtotal or total maxillectomy defects presents a significant challenge to the maxillofacial prosthodontist[43-46]. Often there is inadequate retention, stability, and support for the prosthesis because of the apparent loss of anatomic structures. Patients with such defects have significant difficulties in swallowing, speech, mastication, and esthetics.[43,44] They often have poor lip support, scarring of the lip, midfacial collapse, lip incompetency, drooping commissures, and trismus due tosurgical morbidities[43,44]. The nose is often collapsed due to loss of nasal septum and anterior nasal spine, resulting in esthetic and breathing difficulties.

Educating the patient about the advantages, disadvantages and understanding patients expectations is the key factor for successful rehabilitation after maxillectomy. For a complete bilateral obturator prosthesis, various methods have been put on such as,

1. Existing anatomic undercuts and lateral scar band[44,46];

2. Remaining maxillary structures, such as the posterior third of the soft palate[46];

3. Titanium hollow reconstruction plate attached to the zygomatic bone[47];

4. Implants placed in the remnant of the maxilla, grafted bone, or distracted bone[45]; and

5. Zygomatic implants[43,48-50].

Pterygoid implant has been defined as "implant placement through the maxillary tuberosity and into the pterygoid plate.[51]" These implants were first introduced by Tulasne in 1989[52,53]. The pterygoid implant originates in the tuberosity region and then follows an oblique mesiocranial direction proceeding posteriorly toward the pyramidal process; it subsequently proceeds upward between both wings of the pterygoid processes and finds its encroachment in the pterygoid or scaphoid fossa of the sphenoid bone[54,55]. The length of these implants ranges from 15 to 20 mm, and they are generally placed at an angle of 458 to 508 to the horizontal plane[53,54]. Usually, a combination of osteotomes and surgical drills with long extensions are used because of the semi-blinded nature of the surgical procedure and the bone density of the pterygoid plates and to minimize the potential for injuring vital structures[54-56]. Though previous reports have advocated the use of general anesthesia for implant placement in this region, more recent reports have described the use of local anesthesia[56,57].

Some of the complications with surgical placement reported in the literature include slight venous bleeding[56], minor trismus[56], misplacement of the implant[55,58], and a unique case of continuous episode of pain and discomfort[59]. A recent case report described the use of a long zygomatic implant in the pterygoid region that resulted in an intracerebral penetration[60]. Careful planning and use of cone-beam computerized tomography imaging may help prevent some of these complications.

Pterygoid implants have been primarily used in the rehabilitation of patients with atrophic maxilla or for purposes of avoiding maxillary sinus augmentation procedures. Only 1 article in the literature has mentioned the use of pterygoid implants in patients undergoing maxillectomy[61]. However, this article did not describe the number of pterygoid implants or the number and type of patients who received these implants. The primary advantage of using pterygoid implants is that the density of bone in this area affords good anchorage potential, which may be superior to that of any other part of the maxilla[52,62]. However, the main disadvantage of this procedure is the technique sensitivity and difficulty in access for clinicians and patients[52,62]. The longterm survival rate of these implants is not well reported but one study depicting survival over a period of up to 10 years calculated a cumulative survival rate of 95.3%.[56]

Other studies have found similar survival rates over a varying time period.[62-64] The purpose of this clinical report is to describe the comprehensive rehabilitation of a patient undergoing bilateral maxillectomy using pterygoid implants for retention and support.

CLINICAL RECOMMENDATIONS

The pterygoid implant is placed in the region of the first or second maxillary molars and follows a diagonal direction posteriorly towards the pyramidal process. The implant ultimately anchors in the pterygoid fossa of the sphenoid bone. The angulation of pterygoid implants ranges from 45°-50° towards the maxillary plane [Bidra 2011].

In clinical reality, whenever pterygoid implants are described those are in reality tuberosity implants with an anchorage in the pterygoid plate and thus the treatment difficulties are very limited. As with every implant surgery the preparation of the implant bed is of high importance and treatment planning should be performed with great attention to the anatomical structures and bone availability/quality.

Due to the presence of type III or IV cancellous bone in this region, a preferred choice of implant type is the Nobel Active implant given its high primary stability in soft bone.

TREATMENT PLANNING CONSIDERATIONS

The predictability of the outcome of an implant restoration in the posterior part of the mouth is dependent on many variables including but not limited to the following:

1. Available space

2. Implant number and position

3. Occlusal considerations

4. Type of prosthesis

5. Overall treatment plan.

Available space

A. Mesiodistal:-

Though aesthetics is secondary in restoring the posterior areas of the oral cavity, care should still be taken with implant position to allow restorations that will be functional and as close to the natural dentition as possible, to allow proper development of occlusion and embrasure forms for patient comfort. Mesiodistal space is evaluated in two dimensions. Adequate prosthetic space must exist to provide the patient with a restoration that mimics natural tooth contours. If inadequate prosthetic space exists, it must be created through enameloplasty of adjacent teeth or orthodontic repositioning. The mesiodistal space required essentially depends on the type of tooth being replaced (molar or premolar), and the number of teeth being replaced. The natural maxillary first and second premolar, and first molar have an average mesiodistal size of 7.1, 6.6 and 10.4 mm respectively. The dimensions of these teeth at the CEJ are 4.8, 4.7 and 7.9 mm. At a distance 2 mm from the CEJ the teeth measure 4.2 mm, 4.1 mm and 7.0

mm[69,70]. Decisions need to be made with regards to implant size. The following guidelines should be used when selecting implant size and evaluating mesiodistal space for implant placement[71]:

1. The implant should be at least 1.5 mm away from the adjacent teeth

2. The implant should be at least 3 mm away from an adjacent implant

3. A wider diameter implant should be selected for molar teeth.

Based on the above for two 4 mm diameter implants a space of 14 mm is required. This amount of space would suffice to replace two premolars. If two premolars and a molar are required an additional space is necessary. This situation can be resolved by placement of two implants and fabrication of an FPD or placement of three implants. In either case a wider diameter implant is required in the molar region (5 mm). If three implants are planned a total space of 23 mm is required. Similar guidelines should be followed when treatment planning implants in the posterior mandible. The size of the prosthetic tooth must be considered when placing implants; the implant must be placed sufficiently away from the adjacent tooth to allow the restorative dentist to develop appropriate contours. If an implant placed for a premolar restoration is placed too close to the adjacent tooth, compromised contours and unnecessary loss of hard and soft tissue adjacent to the implant result. Placing the restoration too far from the adjacent tooth also results in unfavourable contours and development of cantilever type forces on the implant.

Planning for a premolar restoration requires the surgeon to place the implant 1.5 mm away from the adjacent root. Molar teeth are wider mesiodistally and for molar implant restorations the implant needs to be placed 2.5 mm away from the adjacent tooth to allow development of appropriate restorative contours.

B. Buccolingual:-

At least 6 mm of bone buccolingually is required for placement of a 4 mm diameter implant and 7 mm for a wider diameter 5 mm implant. The implants should be placed so that the projection of the fixture is contained within the anticipated crown form. The screw access should be positioned towards the centre of the occlusal surface. Posterior mandibular fixtures should be placed so that the exit angle of the screw access should point towards the inner incline of the palatal cusp. Posterior maxillary implants should be placed so that the exit angle of the screw access points towards the inner incline of the buccal cusp. Correct angulation is always achieved if the surgeon is diligent and makes use of a surgical guide to place implants in the correct position. Placing implants in off angle positions always complicates the process for the restorative dentist who now has to use a host of restorative components to achieve an acceptable end result.

C. Occlusogingival:- This parameter also needs to be considered in two dimensions:

1. Adequate space for restoration

2. Adequate osseous volume for placement of the implant.

Adequate space for restoration

Sufficient space must exist to allow the restorative dentist to fabricate restorations which are harmonious aesthetically with the adjacent teeth. On examination the space between the residual ridge and the opposing occlusal plane should be evaluated. Replacing premolar and molar teeth requires 10 mm of space between the residual ridge and the opposing occlusion. 7 mm would be considered the bare minimum. Often, when teeth are missing for prolonged periods of time, opposing teeth overerupt and compromise the restorative space. If this is minimal, enameloplasty or minimal restorative therapy may be required to create space. On occasion molar teeth over-erupt to the extent that they contact the opposing residual ridge. Orthodontic intrusion of these teeth is a technique-sensitive procedure which requires diligence from both the surgeon and orthodontist. Options include both elective endodontics, crown lengthening and preparation of the tooth for a full coverage restoration. In instances where the root trunk is short, consideration must be given to extraction and implant replacement as an alternative so that sufficient space can be created. Often when space is limited towards the posterior quadrant the patient must be informed that it may not be possible to fabricate restorations to replace all of their missing teeth.

Adequate osseous volume for placement of the implant

Often the clinician is confronted with single tooth gaps that present all of the pre-requisites for successful implant therapy, with the exception of sufficient vertical bone height. The question arises: what is the minimal height of the implant required to support a posterior restoration? Clinicians have anecdotally used the longest implant possible, being concerned with the ratio between the implant and suprastructure length

— the thought process being that an unfavourable implant:suprastructure ratio will cause crestal bone resorption. There are data from prospective multicentre studies to show that shorter implants of 6-8 mm did not show increased crestal bone loss in comparison to longer implants (10-12 mm) and the unfavourable ratio between the implant and the supra structure did not lead to more pronounced crestal bone resorption[72,73].

For a standard protocol 7.5 mm of bone height is required for a 6 mm long fixture and 8.5 mm is required for a 7 mm fixture. Prior to fixture placement the maxillary sinus, inferior alveolar canal and mental foramina must be evaluated by means of a CT scan. There should be at least 2 mm of bone between the apical end of the implant and neurovascular structures. Advances in onlay grafting, distraction osteogenesis and maxillary sinus augmentation allow the surgeon to place implants in sites which were previously contraindicated[74-76].

Sinus augmentation provides adequate bone volume to place implants but does not correct for vertical space deficiencies. The patient must be aware that prosthetically, long teeth with root form or pink porcelain will be required. The diameter of the implant also plays a role in occluso-gingival placement. Originally wider diameter implants were created as a rescue implant for conditions in which the standard 3.75 mm implant could not be stabilised. For the restorative dentist the wide diameter implant has been a welcome addition. The improved stability, greater surface area and improved force distribution are particular benefits in the posterior part of the mouth where forces are greater. The success with wide diameter implants replacing molar teeth has been documented in clinical studies[77]. Certainly the wider diameter implants come closer to replicating the emergence profile of the molar tooth.

With regards to placement, use of a standard 4 mm diameter implant for a molar tooth requires the implant to be placed slightly deeper so that an appropriate emergence profile can be developed. The limiting factor in placement may be vital structures, in which case the prosthesis design will require the contours to extend horizontally from the implant. Maintaining hygiene becomes very difficult and some patients may even complain of food entrapment. Use of wider diameter implants allows shallower placement of the implant since the transition in emergence profile from the wider diameter is not as pronounced. Clinicians have also advocated placement of two implants in molar positions to compensate for poor bone quality[78]. Double implants more closely mimic the anatomy of the roots being replaced and double the anchorage surface area.

Other advantages include eliminations of antero-posterior cantilever, reduction of rotational forces exerted and reduction of screw loosening. However, daily oral hygiene may be more difficult and a major limitation in placing two implants is insufficient mesiodistal space.

Implant number and position

The number of implants to be placed depends on the quality and quantity of bone. When three posterior teeth are missing, two or three implants may be required. It is preferred to place three implants in the maxilla because it is a less dense bone. This is because even if one of the implants fail the dentist may still continue with the previously planned prosthesis.

Cantilever type prosthesis failed due to the mechanical complications of the abutment teeth. Abutments can be modified in length and taper and the connector size can also be modified to obtain maximum strength.

Cantiliever forwards is prepared.

Wider implants are preferred. Buccally facing implants have advantage.

In cases where bone volume is not enough there are two options: either a bone augmentation procedure or a simple approach of cantilevering.

When cantileevering the occlusal surface of the cantilever should be minimum so that majority of the load is distributed along the long axis of the implants. Distal cantilevers are more unfavourable from a biomechanical point of view and have more complications. the decision of choosing between either two implants or three implants depends upon how the load is distributed[79].

Practically placing three implants in an absolute linear arrangement is difficult and there is a certain degree of tripoding that occurs. If only two implants are placed, using a wider diameter implant will be equally beneficial as of the non- linear configuration[79].

Occlusal considerations

The masticatory forces developed by a patient with implants is equal to that of natural dentition[80]. A general assessment of the amount of load likely to be placed on the implant should be done prior. A patient with bruxism should be provided with more number of implants to compensate the load. Analysis of the bone density and volume, anticipated loads and planned restorative design should be done prior to determination of length and diameter of the implant. The range of motion of osseointegrated implants has been reported to be approximately 3-5 microns. Displacement of a tooth begins with an initial phase of periodontal compliance that is non-linear and complex, followed by a secondary movement phase occurring with the engagement of the alveolar bone. In contrast, an implant deflects in a linear and elastic pattern and movement of the implant under load is dependent on elastic deformation of the bone.

Techniques should be used to minimise excessive loading on implant supported restorations. There should be no contact of posterior teeth on both working and non- working sides. Initial occlusal contact should occur on the natural dentition. Cuspal inclinations on implant supported restorations should also be shallower. Any type of cantilever force should be minimised, which includes anterior, posterior and buccolingual cantilever. In cases where there has been extreme resorption of the maxillary bone, teeth are set in a cross bite relationship to minimise offset loads. When multiple posterior teeth are replaced splinting of the implants can be done.[80,81,82,83]

The stress distribution can be manipulated by splinting. Splinting also has practical advantages like there are fewer proximal contacts to adjust.

Type of prosthesis

Screw retained or cemented

Screw retained prosthesis have the advantage of retrievability. This facilitates individual implant evaluation along with soft tissue inspection. Also shade changing, repair and maintaining oral hygiene becomes easy with the prosthesis can be easily unscrewed. On the other hand cemented prosthesis provide more esthetic appearance. A cemented prosthesis may require sectioning to tighten a loose abutment[85].

Whether screw retained or cemented-n this depends upon the tooth being replaced. For instance the occlusal surface of a premolar is small and patients may object to occlusal access holes in restorations replacing the first and second premolar. These restorations may be designed to be cement retained. When using cement retained restorations they should be designed to follow the contours of the gingiva The margin of the abutment should also be kept as minimally subgingival as aesthetics will allow. Placing a cement margin too deep will cause difficulty in removal of excess cement[84].

Splinted or non-splinted

Stress distribution can be manipulated by splinting[84]. There is an increase in the retention of the prosthesis with increase in the number of splinted abutments. Splinting reduces the risk of screw loosening and unretained restorations. When more than three units are splinted sectioning and soldering will be required to improve fit.

Abutment level vs. implant level restoration, segmented vs. non-segmented

When implants are aligned to allow screw retention, unless the soft tissue depth is more than 3 mm, implant supported restorations are almost always restored directly to the implant. Screw retained abutments are only used when the implants are placed deeply or soft tissue depth is more. In some cases a titanium interface is desired and in these situations abutments can be selected to allow a supra mucosal restorative interface. The only disadvantages of this is that there will be a display of metal on the restoration. Sometimes screw retained pre-angled abutments are required. when these are to be used the implant must be placed deeper to accommodate the thickness of the abutment[85]. When cemented restorations are used the abutments placed should match the transitional contours required to allow proper contour of the restorations. The cement margin should not be placed more than 1 mm sub mucosal to facilitate cement removal. When cement retention is desired there must be sufficient inter occlusal space.

Overall treatment plan

In cases of long span fixed partial dentures there should be fewer number of pontics and more number of implant abutments. The use implants should be based on prosthetically oriented risk assessment. Prosthetically oriented risk assessment involves comprehensive evaluation of potential abutment teeth.

SURGICAL PROCEDURE

The literature describes 2 different anatomic locations where pterygoid implants are placed: the pterygoid process and the pterygomaxillary region. These are frequently not clearly distinguished by authors; however, because of the differences between these locations, different implant-placement techniques should be used.

Implants are inserted in the pterygoid process using a technique that requires surgical experience and detailed knowledge of anatomy of the area. The implant is anchored in the pterygoid plate of the sphenoid bone, through the maxillary and palatine bones and with distal angulation between 358 and 558, depending on the maxillary sinus floor and the height of the bone of the tuberosity. The internal maxillary artery crosses 1 cm above the pterygopalatine suture as it enters the pterygopalatine fossa. Therefore, the distance from the artery to the lower end of the pterygomaxillary suture is 25 mm. Because of the absence of vital structures in the insertion area, it is a safe working area for the surgeon. Any bleeding in this region will be from the veins of the pterygoid muscle, and it can be stopped quickly once the intraosseous fixation is inserted and will not restart once the implant is stabilized. The implant site is prepared combining drills and straight osteotomes, according the technique described by Valero 'n et al used by other researchers. The entry point is determined with a round bur. Preparation of the implant bed then starts with the smallest straight osteotome, followed by a pilot drill to establish the direction of the implant axis. Preparation continues with consecutive cylindricosteotomes in combination with drills of increasing diameter.

Implants in the pterygomaxillary region are placed within the maxillary tuberosity, near or parallel to the posterior wall of the sinus. The surgical procedure is similar to that of implants anchored in the pterygoid process, the only difference being the use of curved instead of straight osteotomes. The angle should 108 to 208 degrees to simulate the proper angulation of the third molar. Bahat et al consider it necessary to open the patient's mouth a minimum of about 35 mm to achieve good implant angulation. The implant site is carved with drills with increasingly larger diameters. However, Valero´n et al recommend the use of osteotomes, which preserve more bone and reduce surgical risks, especially hemorrhages. Nocini et al used anatomically modified osteotomes to facilitate access to the maxillary tuberosity area. Pen arrocha et al combined burs and osteotomes to place 68 implants pterygomaxillary region in 45 patients, thus joining the advantages of the 2 techniques: osteotomes minimize surgical risk, preserve more bone, and allow more (tactile) control/feel in such an inaccessible area, whereas drills facilitate the creation of the bed, especially in the dense cortical bone area.

COMPLICATIONS

One of the major surgical risks that may occur during the surgery is bleeding,

1. Because of the proximity of the internal maxillary artery, which runs 1 cm above the pterygomaxillary suture; this complication is rare, is not mentioned in most studies. Valero ´n and Valero ´n

2. Described a minor venous bleeding caused by the insertion of the drill a few millimeters into the retropterygoid area. It was resolved with local hemostatic methods.

Krekmanov14 reported problems when anchoring the implants into the pterygoid process. An implant was lost during placement due to drilling beyond the pterygoid process. Vrielinck et al lost 4 of 6 implants due to problems in placing them in the initially drilled implant bed and having to place them in a different position, which resulted in insufficient bone anchorage.

SUCCESS RATE

The success of implants was assessed using Albrektsson's and Buser's clinical and radiologic criteria. The weighted average success of pterygoid implants was 90.7%. Balshi et al reported 3 clinical series of pterygoid implants.

In 1995, they made a preliminary study in which 51 pterygoid implants with machined surface were placed in 41 patients with a follow-up period of 1–63 months. The success rate was 86.3%. In 1999, they increased the sample to 356 implants, obtaining a success rate of 88.2% with a follow-up of 54 months. In 2005, they placed 164 pterygoid implants with treated surfaces and, after 54 months of follow-up, observed a success rate that was statistically significantly higher than in previous studies (96.3%).

Vrielinck et al placed 14 pterygomaxillary implants and had a success rate of 71% after an average follow-up of 6–24 months. The failures occurred because the implants did not follow the drilled bed and were therefore out of place.

Ridelletal reported a 100% success after placing 22 implants in the maxillary tuberosity area and after a follow-up of 12 years.

Accuracy using zygoma and pterygoid implants was reported in two papers. The length of these implants is three to four times that of a standard oral implant. This means that even slight angular deviations may lead to important deviations at the extremity. In one ex vivo study, 24 six zygoma fixtures with a length of 45 mm were planned in three cadaver heads using a custom made bone-supported drilling with intimate fitting to the underlying jawbone. In four of the six implants, the angle between the placed and the planned implants was less than 3°. The largest deviation noted was 6.9° resulting in a measurable deviation of 6.74 mm in craniocaudal direction at the apex of the implant. This was explained by the fact that a metal cylinder came loose during the surgery. A clinical study reported on 29 cases with zygoma, pterygoid and standard oral implants using bone supported guides. The osteotomies were performed using only two drills with corresponding guide sleeves but the fixtures were manually installed without the guide. After implant surgery, a postoperative CT scan was taken of 12 randomly selected patients to be matched with the preoperative planning and the deviations were calculated. For the zygoma implants, the maximum deviation was 7.4 mm coronally (mean 2.8 mm), 9.7 mm apically (mean 4.5 mm), and 9.0° for the angular deviation (mean 5.1°). For the standard implants installed the maximum deviation was 4.7 mm (mean 1.51 mm) coronally and 6.4 mm (mean 3.07 mm) apically. The pterygoid implants deviated on average 3.57 mm (range 0.2–7.8) at the entry point and 7.77 mm (range 1.1–16.1) at the exit point. The average axis deviation was 10.18° (range 1.7°–18.0°). Probably because of the substantial deviations from the planning disappointing cumulative implant survivals were reported, two zygoma implants (7% failures) and four pterygoid implants (29% failures) were lost because of this misplacement. Six standard implants were lost (8% failures) because no initial implant stability was achieved at the time of surgery. The author explained that all patients suffered from severe atrophy of the maxillary bone and had a low bone quality according to the Misch classification. Furthermore, manual fixture installation may have imposed an extra risk for additional misplacement. Summarizing the scrutinized papers regarding zygoma and pterygoid implants, one can conclude that the overall coronal, apical, or angular deviation is, respectively, 2.56 mm, 3.7 mm and 3.92°. In conclusion, it can be stated that only 10 publications compared the preoperative implant planning with the postoperative implant locations. Hence very few papers evaluated accuracy of computer guided stereolithographic surgery in a scientifically objective way. All data published indicate that a substantial deviation is found between virtually planned and in vivo placed implants. Enlarging a stiff surface for guide positioning improves the accuracy, although bone-supported guides are less accurate than teeth-supported ones. Although flapless surgery is quite often used in daily practice, very few papers on accuracy are available when using stereolithographic mucosal-supported surgical guides for full jaw rehabilitation in maxilla or mandible. Additionally, the study designs reporting on different supporting surfaces (dental and mucosal), different implant systems or designs (standard oral implants and zygoma/ pterygoid implants) and the rather limited number of implants included in the papers lead to the conclusion that the evidence on accuracy is lacking.

PTERYGOID IMPLANTS VERSUS ZYGOMATIC IMPLANTS

	PTERYGOID IMPLANTS	ZYGOMATIC IMPLANTS
Type of implants	Single piece Implants is used. No screw loosening and no crestal bone loss.	Screw based implants used. Screw loosening is a problem
Cantilevers	No cantilevers placed	Molars if given are placed as cantilevers, which decrease the life of the bridge and cause screw loosening on the implant.
Criteria	No contraindications	Symptom free and pathologically free sinus
Relative risk of failure	Since sinus is not involved, no risk of sinusitis	Risk of sinus infection
Permanent bridge	Permanent ceramic bridge on 3rd day of implant placement, as the implant engages hard cortical bone.	Acrylic/plastic for first 4 months. Then cantilever permanent ceramic bridge given after 4 months.
CT scan	Not needed.	Compulsorily needed

Anaesthesia	Local anaesthesia with or without sedation	General anaesthesia
Surgical guide	Not needed	Compulsorily needed
Cost of implant	Being regular sized single piece implant it is relatively cheap.	Zygomatic implants are very long manufactured specifically for the purpose, hence very expensive. Cost of the technique is more as CT scan and surgical guide is used.
No of implants for full upper jaw	8-10 for upper jaw.	6 -10 for upper jaw
No of teeth	14 teeth are given. Teeth replaced till second molar	10 teeth or 12 teeth given. 2nd molar is not given.
No of trips	One trip, as permanent ceramic crown or bridge is placed in 3 days	Two trips. Permanent teeth fixed after 3 months of implant placement.
Warranty	Lifetime warranty on implant	No warranty

RECENT ADVANCES

The maxillofacial treatment of advanced crest atrophy with two stage surgery is an invasive procedure. During the healing period, removable temporaries are recommended. Therefore, a rather long period is necessary to support the edentulous arch with a fixed aesthetic restoration on the implants. One surgery is necessary with the concept of oral implantology presented here. Without bone grafting and mandibular nerve repositioning, it is less invasive. Also, immediate implantation has favourable results. The procedure is a low trauma surgery. By application of immediate functional loading on the disk design implants 7 to 8 days after implantation, both arches are already equipped with fixed aesthetic temporaries. With a correct implant technique to achieve tricortical or multicortical support, this procedure is safe, less invasive, and decreases chair time.

Disk Implants

The advantages of disk design implants are based on several significant facts:

1) The loading transmission interface is mainly around the basal disks;

2) Initial stability is achieved by anchoring the disks in the cortical bone;

3) The density of laminar bone and the residual bone height are not as

important as with root-form implants.

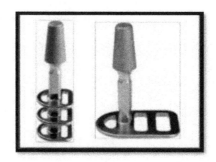

Implant success with 5 mm of available alveolar bone height is possible. The thickness of the disks is 0.5 mm. Therefore, the placement of Disc implants allows for primary bone healing in the area around the disks (principle of fracture healing). The posterior zones of the mandible are not rigid bone structures in movement but are flexible. Disc implants are not rigid either. The flexibility of this implant form (especially Mono disk implants with a long shaft) adjusts physiologically to the functional demands on the mandible.

Immediate Function Implants

Today, modern implant design and the use of 3D CAT Scans allow experienced dental professionals to insert the implants, and immediately place the new teeth on the implants. Research has shown that when properly applied, this one-stage approach results in as good or better implant success rates as the traditional two-stage approach.

Benefits of Immediate Function

- Shortened treatment time (it is possible to go from tooth loss to having functional and aesthetic teeth in one treatment session),
- Better clinical efficiency,
- Greater patient comfort,

- The elimination of bone grafts and sinus lifts, and

- Patients always leave with teeth!

All – on – 4 Implant

- The All-on-4 Dental Implant Procedure uses four implants, with the back implants angulated to take maximum advantage of existing bone.

- Special implants also were developed that could support the immediate fitting of replacement teeth.

- This treatment is attractive to those with dentures or in need of full upper and/or lower restorations.

- With the All-on-4 Procedure, qualified patients receive just four implants and a full set of new replacement teeth in just one appointment—without bone grafts!

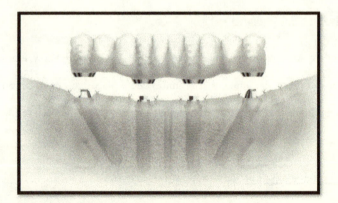

- All four titanium implants are placed so that the bone will

  grow around and secure them in place

- With only four implants, there is much less invasive and

  lengthy surgery.

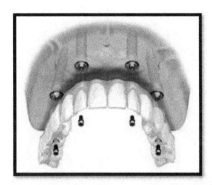

- Once the implants are in place, the Oral Surgeon attaches abutments to which the new replacement teeth can be secured.
- The Prosthodontist fits the replacement teeth on the abutments and adjusts the bite for comfort and a beautiful smile.

<u>Interdenatal Esthetics</u>

- A number of cases show deficiency of papilla in the interdental papilla between the implant or between implants and teeth, which poses an esthetic problem.

- This is counteracted by injection of hyaluronic acid, commonly available as Restylane.

- Its effect lasts for 6 – 24 months after which a new dose is administered.

SUMMARY AND CONCLUSION

The posterior maxilla has been described as the most difficult and problematic intraoral area confronting the implant practitioner, requiring a maximum of ingenuity for the achievement of successful results[86,87]. Solutions like sinus lifts often involve double site procedures and added bone grafting that involves a longer healing period, possibility of perforation of the sinus membrane along with the risk of infection[88].

In such cases, when patients have severely atrophic maxilla and are unwilling or unable to undergo extensive bone grafting, various newer treatment modalities like zygomatic and pterygoid implants were introduced.

Pterygoid and Zygoma implants provide a solution for a patient with a severely resorbed jaw bone with minimal surgical trauma and maximum oral function. The zygomaticus implant is an alternative to bone grafting into the sinus area. The implants can be placed in better quality bone, which establishes stable anchorage for non-removable teeth.

These implants are indicated in the cases which have insufficient bone but want an implant supported prosthesis. These implants can be placed in severely resorbed jaw bone with minimal surgical trauma and maximum oral function. These implants can be an alternative to sinus lift procedure for indicated cases. The implants can be placed in better quality bone, which establishes stable anchorage for non-removable teeth.

Due to both the anatomical intricacies of the zygomatic bone and the implant length, the placement of zygoma implants still represents a challenge to prosthodontists. To minimize the risks of surgery, 3D reconstruction, preoperative planning, registration, surgical implant guidance, and a motion tracking algorithm should be used.

The posteriorly placed maxillary implant have been described as tuberosity implants[89-91]pterygoid plate implants[92], and pterygomaxillary implants[93]. The varied terminology arises as a result of the various anatomic structures that may be engaged in the placement of implants in this region. The precise structures offering potential support for implant placement are the tuberosity of the maxillary bone, the pyramidal process of the palatine bone, and the pterygoid process of the sphenoid bone[94]. Zygomatic implants and recorded a high survival rate which is about 98.4–100 % and for pterygoid implants success rate ranges between 88 -95% .

Such implants have provided successful support for a variety of prosthesis forms, including multi-implant complete arch fixed prostheses, complete removable over dentures with fixed retention bars, multiple implant s upported restorations. Because of the anatomic factors and some biomechanical factors[97], one would expect the success rate for implants placed into the posterior maxilla to be lower than that for other locations.

These implants are also notable for their length, being much longer than standard implants: zygomatic and pterygoid implants are approximately 30 to 55 mm and 15 to 20 mm long respectively. The length necessary to ensure anchorage to the bone.

- The main feature of these implants is that they are placed on two bones that never undergo resorption, even with severe atrophy of the jawbone: the zygomatic bone, or cheekbone, in the case of zygomatic implants, and the pterygoid bone in the case of pterygoid implants. This surgical technique therefore offers a good alternative to the placement of bone grafts in the case of significant maxillary resorption, and also reduces treatment time in a way that is safe, quick, and comfortable for the patient. On some occasions, the placement of these implants is accompanied by the use of standard implants, depending on the amount of bone the patient has.

- Appropriate case selection, good occlusal harmony, careful management of hard and soft tissues, and maintainence of oral hygiene all contribute the success and predictability of dental implants.

BIBLIOGRAPHY

1. Bedrossian E, Stumpel L,Beckely M, Indersana T. The zygomatic implant: preliminary data on treatment of severely resorbed maxillae. A clinical report. Int J Oral Maxillofac Implants 2002;17:861–5.

2. Bedrossian E, Stumpel L J .Immediate stabilization at stage II of zygomatic implants :rationale and technique. J Prosthet Dent 2001;86:10–4.

3. Stella JP, Warner MR. Sinus slot technique for simplification and improved orientation of zygomaticus dental implants: a technical note . Int J Oral Maxillofac Implants 2000; 15: 889–93.

4. Parel SM, Brånemark PI,OhrnellLO,Svensson B. Remote implant anchorage for the rehabilitation of maxillary defects. J Prosthet Dent 2001;86:377–81.

5. Higuchi KW.The zygomaticus fixture:an alternative approach for implant anchorage in the posterior maxilla. Ann R AustralasColl Dent Surg 2000;15:28–33.

6. Schnitman PA, Wohrle PS, RubensteinJE,et al. Ten-year results for Brånemark implants immediately loaded with fixed prostheses at implant placement. Int J Oral Maxillofac Implants 1997;12:495–503.

7. Jaffin RA, Kumar A, Bermann CL. Immediate loading of implants in partially and fully edentulous jaws: a series of 27 case reports. J Periodontol 2000;71:833–5.

8. Salama H, Rose LF, Salama M, Betts NH. Immediate ofbilaterally splinted titanium root-form implants in prosthodontics – a technique reexamined: two cases. Int J Periodontol Rest Dent 1995;15:344–60.

9. Tarnow DP, Emtiaz S, Classi A. Immediate loading of threaded implants at stage 1 surgery in edentulous arches: ten consecutive case reports with 1- to 5-year data. Int J Oral Maxillofac Implants 1997;12:319–24.

10. Zhao R, SkalakR, Brånemark PI. An analysis of a fixed prosthesis supported by the zygomatic fixture. (In press).

11. Parel SM. The single-piece milled titanium implant bridge. Dent Today 2003;21:106–8.

12. J. Claveroand S. Lundgren, Ramus or chin grafts for maxillary sinus inlay and local onlay augmentation: comparison of donor site morbidity and complications," Clinical Implant Dentistry and Related Research,vol.5, no.3,pp. 154–160,2003.

13. M. J. Yaremchuk, "Vascularized bone grafts for maxillofacial reconstruction," Clinics in Plastic Surgery, vol. 16, pp. 29–39, 1989.

14. M.Sj¨ostr¨om,L.Sennerby,H.Nilson,andS.Lundgren,"Reconstructionoftheatrophiceden tulousmaxillawithfreeiliaccrest grafts and implants: a 3-year report of a prospective clinical study," Clinical Implant Dentistry and Related Research, vol. 9, no.1,pp.46–59,2007.

15. L. K. Cheung, Q. Zhang, Z. G. Zhang, and M. C. M. Wong, "Reconstruction of maxillectomy defect by transport distraction osteogenesis,"International Journal of Oral and Maxillofacial Surgery, vol.32 ,no.5, pp.515–522, 2003.

16. E. Nystr¨om, H. Nilson, J. Gunne, and S. Lundgren, "Reconstruction of the atrophic maxilla with interpositional bone grafting/Le Fort I osteotomy and endosteal implants: a 11–16 year follow-up," International Journal of Oral and Maxillofacial Surgery, vol.38, no.1, pp.1–6, 2009.

17. R. G. Triplett and S. R. Schow, "Autologous bone grafts and endosseous implants: complementary techniques," Journal of OralandMaxillofacialSurgery,vol.54,no.4,pp.486–494,1996.

18. M. Del Fabbro, T. Testori, L. Francetti, and R. Weinstein, "Systematic review of survival rates for implants placed in the grafted maxillary sinus," International Journal of Periodontics andRestorativeDentistry,vol.24,no.6,pp.565–577,2004.

19. L. Vrielinck, C. Politis, S. Schepers, M. Pauwels, and I. Naert, "Image-based planning and clinical validation of zygoma and pterygoid implant placement in patients with severe   bone atrophyusingcustomizeddrillguides.Preliminaryresultsfromaprospectiveclinicalfollow-upstudy,"InternationalJournalof   OralandMaxillofacialSurgery,vol.32,no.1,pp.7–14,2003.

20. K. Lal, G. S. White, D. N. Morea, and R. F. Wright, "Use of stereolithographic templates for surgical and prosthodontic implant planning and placement. Part I. The concept," Journal ofProsthodontics,vol.15,no.1,pp.51–58,2006.

21. R.Ewers, K.Schicho, G.Undtetal., "Basicresearchand 12 years of clinical experience incomputer-assisted navigation technology: a review," International Journal of Oral and Maxillofacial Surgery,vol.34,no.1,pp.1–8,2005.

22. L.R.Duarte, H.N.Filho, C.E.Francischone, L.G.Peredo,and P. I. Br°anemark, "The establishment of a protocol for the total rehabilitation of atrophic maxillae employing four zygomatic fixtures in an immediate loading system—a 30-month clinical and radiographic   follow-up,"   Clinical   Implant   Dentistry   and RelatedResearch,vol.9,no.4,pp.186–196,2007.

23. P. Mal´o, M. de Araujo Nobre, and I .Lopes, "A new approach to rehabilitate the severely atrophic maxilla using extra maxillary anchored implants inimmediate function : apilotstudy," Journal of Prosthetic Dentistry,vol.100,no.5,pp.354–366,2008.

24. M. Sti'evenart and C. Malevez, "Rehabilitation of totally atrophied maxilla by means of four zygomatic implants and fixed prosthesis: a 6-40-month follow-up," International Journal of OralandMaxillofacialSurgery,vol.39,pp.358–363,2010.

25. B. Al-Nawas, J. Wegener, C. Bender, and W. Wagner, "Critical soft tissue parameters of the zygomatic implant," Journal of ClinicalPeriodontology,vol.31,no.7,pp.497–500,2004.

26. M. Sti'evenart and C. Malevez, "Rehabilitation of totally atrophied maxilla by means of four zygomatic implants and fixed prosthesis: a 6-40-month follow-up," International Journal of OralandMaxillofacialSurgery,vol.39,pp.358–363,2010.

27. J. P. Becktor, S. Isaksson, P. Abrahamsson, and L. Sennerby, "Evaluation of 31 zygomatic implants and 74 regular dental implants used in 16 patients for prosthetic reconstruction of the atrophic maxilla with cross – arch fixed bridges, "Clinical Implant Dentistry and Related Research, vol.7 ,no.3 ,pp.159–165,2005.

28. C. Malevez, M. Abarca, F. Durdu, and P. Daelemans, "Clinical outcome of 103 consecutive zygomatic implants: a 6-48 months follow- upstudy," Clinical Oral Implants Research,vol.15,no.1, pp.18–22,2004.

29. J.P.Urgell, V. R. Guti'errez, and C. G. Escoda, "Rehabilitation of atrophic maxilla: a review of 101 zygomatic implants, "MedicinaOral, Patologia Oral y Cirugia Bucal, vol. 13, no. 6, Article ID 10489698,pp.E363–E370,2008.

30. C.A. Landes, "Zygoma implant-supported midfacial prosthetic rehabilitation: a 4-year follow-up study including assessment of quality of life, "Clinical Oral ImplantsResearch,vol.16,no.3,pp. 313–325,2005.

31. M. Pe narrocha,C.Carrillo, A.Boronat, and E.Mart'ı, "Level of satisfaction in patients with maxillary full-arch fixed prostheses: zygomatic versus conventional implants,

"International Journal of Oral and Maxillofacial Implants, vol. 22, no. 5, pp. 769–773, 2007.

32. Introducing Dental Implants - John A. Hobkirk, Roger M. Watson, Lloyd Searson

33. Peterson; The Zygoma Implant Sterling R.Schow,DMD; Stephen M.Parel,DDS.pp235

34. The glossary of prosthodontic terms. J Prosthet Dent. 2005; 94:50–52.

35. Ohngren L. Malignant tumors of the maxillo-ethmoidal region. Acta Otolarynogol. 1933;19:476.

36. Sakai S, Fuchihata H, Hamasaki Y. Treatment policy for maxillary sinus carcinoma. ActaOtolaryngol. 1976;82:172–181.

37. Aramany MA. Basic principles of obturator design for partially edentulous patients. Part I: classification. J Prosthet Dent. 1978;40:554–557.

38. Earley MJ. Primary maxillary reconstruction after cancer excision. Br J Plast Surg. 1989;42:628–637.

39. Spiro RH, Strong EW, Shah JP. Maxillectomy and its classification. Head Neck. 1997;19:309–314.

40. Brown JS, Rogers SN, McNally DN, Boyle M. A modified classification for the maxillectomy defect. Head Neck. 2000;22:17– 26.

41. Cordeiro PG, Santamaria E. A classification system and algorithm for reconstruction of maxillectomy and midfacial defects. PlastReconstr Surg. 2000;105:2331–2346.

42. Okay DJ, Genden E, Buchbinder D, Urken M. Prosthodontic guidelines for surgical reconstruction of the maxilla: a classification system of defects. J Prosthet Dent. 2001;86:352–363.

43. Uckan S, Oguz Y, Uyar Y, Ozyesil A. Reconstruction of a total maxillectomy defect with a zygomatic implant-retained obturator. J Craniofac Surg. 2005;16:485–489.

44. Cheng AC, Somerville DA, Wee AG. Altered prosthodontic treatment approach for bilateral complete maxillectomy: a clinical report. J Prosthet Dent. 2004;92:120–124.

45. Oh WS, Roumanas E. Dental implant-assisted prosthetic rehabilitation of a patient with a bilateral maxillectomy defect secondary to mucormycosis. J Prosthet Dent. 2006;96:88–95.

46. Ortegon SM, Martin JW, Lewin JS. A hollow delayed surgical obturator for a bilateral subtotal maxillectomy patient: a clinical report. J Prosthet Dent. 2008;99:14–18.

47. Sjo ̈vall L, Lindqvist C. Hallikainen D. A new method of reconstruction in a patient undergoing bilateral total maxillectomy. Int J Oral Maxillofac Surg. 1992;21:342–345.

48. Parel SM, Bra ˚nemark PI, Ohrnell LO, Svensson B. Remote implant anchorage for the rehabilitation of maxillary defects. J Prosthet Dent. 2001;86:377–381.

49. Schmidt BL, Pogrel MA, Young CW, Sharma A. Reconstruction of extensive maxillary defects using zygomaticus implants. J Oral Maxillofac Surg. 2004;62:82–89.

50. Tamura H, Sasaki K, Watahiki R. Primary insertion of implants in the zygomatic bone following subtotal maxillectomy. Bull Tokyo Dent Coll. 2000;41:21–24.

51. Laney WR. Glossary of Oral and Maxillofacial Implants. Chicago, Ill: Quintessence Publishing; 2007.

52. Tulasne JF. Implant treatment of missing posterior dentition. In: Albrektsson T, Zarb GA, eds. The Branemark Osseointegrated Implant. Chicago, Ill: Quintessence Publishing; 1989;103–108.

53. Tulasne JF. Osseointegrated fixtures in the pterygoid region. In: Worthington P, Branemark PI, eds. Advanced Osseointegration Surgery: Applications in the Maxillofacial Region. Chicago, Ill: Quintessence Publishing; 1992;182–188.

54. Graves SL. The pterygoid plate implant: a solution for restoring the posterior maxilla. Int J PeriodontRestor Dent. 1994;14: 512–523.

55. Vrielinck L, Politis C, Schepers S, Pauwels M, Naert I. Imagebased planning and clinical validation of zygoma and pterygoid implant placement in patients with severe bone atrophy using customized drill guides. Preliminary results from a prospective clinical follow-up study. Int J Oral Maxillofac Surg. 2003;32:7–14.

56. Valero ´n JF, Valero ´n PF. Long-term results in placement of screw-type implants in the pterygomaxillary-pyramidal region. Int J Oral Maxillofac Implants. 2007;22:195–200.

57. Pen ˜arrocha M, Uribe R, Garcı ´a B, Martı ´ E. Zygomatic implants using the sinus slot technique: clinical report of a patient series. Int J Oral Maxillofac Implants. 2005;20:788–792.

58. Krekmanov L. Placement of posterior mandibular and maxillary implants in patients with severe bone deficiency: a clinical report of procedure. Int J Oral Maxillofac Implants. 2000;15:722–730.

59. Balshi TJ, Lee HY, Hernandez RE. The use of pterygomaxillary implants in the partially edentulous patient: a preliminary report. Int J Oral Maxillofac Implants. 1995;10:89–98.

60. Reychler H, Olszewski R. Intracerebral penetration of a zygomatic dental implant and consequent therapeutic dilemmas: case report. Int J Oral Maxillofac Implants. 2010;25:416–418.

61. Roumanas ED, Nishimura RD, Davis BK, Beumer J III. Clinical evaluation of implants retaining edentulous maxillary obturator prostheses. J Prosthet Dent. 1997;77:184–190.

62. Balshi TJ, Wolfinger GJ. Analysis of 356 pterygomaxillary implants in edentulous arches for fixed prosthesis anchorage. Int J Oral Maxillofac Implants. 1999;14:398–406.

63. Balshi SF, Wolfinger GJ, Balshi TJ. Analysis of 164 titanium oxide-surface implants in completely edentulous arches for fixed prosthesis anchorage using the pterygomaxillary region. Int J Oral Maxillofac Implants. 2005;20:946–952.

64. Pen ˜arrocha M, Carrillo C, Boronat A, Pen ˜arrocha M. Retrospective study of 68 implants placed in the pterygomaxillary region using drills and osteotomes. Int J Oral Maxillofac Implants. 2009;24:720–726.

65. Paprocki GJ, Jacob RF, Kramer DC. Seal integrity of hollow bulb obturators. Int J Prosthodont. 1990;3:457–462.

66. Sakuraba M, Kimata Y, Ota Y, et al. Simple maxillary reconstruction using free tissue transfer and prostheses. Plast Reconstr Surg. 2003;111: 594–598.

67. Chiapasco M, Biglioli F, Autelitano L, Romeo E, Brusati R. Clinical outcome of dental implants placed in fibula-free flaps used for the reconstruction of maxillo-mandibular defects following ablation for tumors or osteoradionecrosis. Clin Oral Implants Res. 2006;17:220–228.

68. Gbara A, Darwich K, Li L, Schmelzle R, Blake F. Long-term results of jaw reconstruction with microsurgical fibula grafts and dental implants. J Oral Maxillofac Surg. 2007;65:1005–1009.

69. Hebel K S, Gajjar R. Achieving superior esthetic results, parameters for implant and abutment selection. Int J Dent Symp 1997; 4: 42-47.

70. Woelfel J B. Dental anatomy: Its relevance to dentistry (4th edn). Philadelphia: Lea and Febiger, 1990.

71. Misch C E. Dental implant prosthetics. pp 281-307. Mosby, 2005.

72. Bischof M, Nedir R, Smukler-Moncler S, Bernard J P. A five year life table analysis of ITI implants. Results from a private practice with emphasis on the use of short implants. Clin Oral Implants Res 2001; 12: 396.

73. Ten Bruggenkate C M, Asikainen P, Foitzik C et al. Short (6 mm) non submerged dental implants: results of a multicenter clinical trial of 1-7 years. Int J Oral Maxillofac Implants 1998; 13: 791-798.

74. Buser D, Von Arx T. Surgical procedures in partially edentulous patients with ITI implants. Clin Oral Implants Res 2000; 11(suppl I): 83-100.

75. Chiapasco M, Abati S, Romeo E, Vogel G. Clinical outcomes of autogenous bone blocks or guided regeneration with a e PTFE membrane for reconstruction of narrow edentulous ridges. Clin Oral Implants Res 1999; 10: 278-288.

76. Chiapasco M, Romeo E, Vogel G. Vertical distraction osteogenesis of edentulous ridges for improvement of oral implant positioning. A clinical report of preliminary results. Int J Oral Maxillofac Implants 2001; 16: 43-51

77. Graves S L, Jansen C E, Siddiqui A A et al. Wide diameter implants, indications, considerations and preliminary results over a two year period. Aust Prosthodont J 1994; 8: 31-37.

78. Balshi T J. First molar replacement with an osseointegrated implant. Quint Int 1990; 21: 61-65.

79. Rangert B, Krough P H J, Langer B, Van Roekel N. Bending overload and implant fracture. A retrospective clinical analysis. Int J Oral Maxillofac Implants 1995; 10: 326-334.

80. CarrA B, Laney W R. Maximum occlusal force levels in patients with osseointegrated oral implant prosthesis and patients with complete dentures. Int J Oral Maxillo fac Implants 1987; 2: 101-108.

81. Sekine M. Problems of occlusion from the standpoint of prosthetic dentistry, with reference to the significance of balanced occlusion in the denture and biological

considerations on the abutment teeth in relation to occlusion pressure in the partial denture. Shikwa Gakuho 1967; 67: 859-867.

82. Schulte W. Implants and the periodontium. Int Dent J 1995; 45: 16-26.

83. Mericske-Stern R, Geering A H, Burgin W B, Graf H. Three dimensional force measurements on mandibular implants supporting overdentures. Int J Oral MaxillofacImplants 1992; 7: 185-194.

84. Cibirka R M, Razoog M E et al. Determining the force absorption quotient for restorative materials used in implant occlusal surfaces. J Prosthet Dent 1992; 67: 361-364.

85. Celletti R, Pameijer C H, Bracchetti G et al. Histologic evaluation of osseointegrated implants restored in non axial functional occlusion with pre-angled abutments. Int J Period Rest Dent 1995; 15: 562-573.

86. Murrah VA (1985) Diabetes mellitus and associated oral manifestations: a review. J Oral Pathol 14:271–281

87. . Cochran DL, Schenk R, Buser D, Wozney JM, Jones AA (1999) Recombinant human bone morphogenetic protein-2 stimulation of bone formation around endosseous dental implants. J Periodontol 70:139–150

88. Balshi TJ, Wolfinger GJ (2000) Management of the posterior maxilla in the compromised patient: historical, current, and future perspectives. Periodontology 33(2003):67–81

89. Bahat O (1992) Osseointegrated implants in the maxillary tuberosity: report on 45 consecutive cases. Int J Oral Maxillofac Implants 7:459–467

90. . Balshi TJ (1992) Single tuberosity osseointegrated implant support for a tissue integrated prosthesis. Int J Periodont Restor Dent 12:345–357

91.. Khayat P, Nader N (1994) The use of osseointegrated implants in the maxillary tuberosity. Pract Periodontics Aesthet Dent 6:53–61

92. Graves SL (1994) The pterygoid plate implant: a solution for restoring the posterior maxilla. Int J PeriodontRestor Dent 14:512–523

93.. Balshi TJ, Hy L, Hernandez RE (1995) The use of pterygomaxillary implants in the partially edentulous patient. Int J Oral Maxillofac Implants 10:89–99

94. Grant JCB (1956) An atlas of anatomy. Williams& Wilkins, Baltimore, p 541

95. Tulasne JF (1992) Implants pterygo-maxillaires experience sur 7 ans. Implant 1(hors serie):39–48

96. Reiser GM (1998) Implant use in the tuberosity, pterygoid, and palatine region anatomic and surgical considerations. In: Nevins M, Mellonig JT (eds) Implant therapy clinical approaches and evidence of success, 2nd edn. Quintessence Books, Chicago

97. Harldson T, Karlsson U, Carlsson GE (1979) Bite force and oral function in complete denture wearers. J Oral Rehabil 6:41–48.

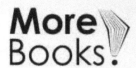
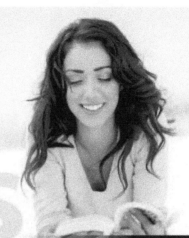
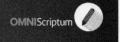